HOW TO BE
SCHOOLGIRL
SKINNY®

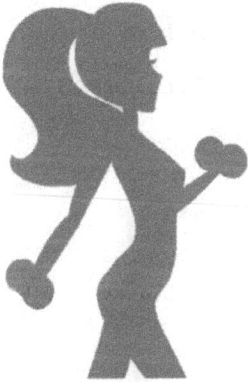

EAT YOUR
CAKE
AND HAVE
YOUR
FIGURE
TOO!

5 WEEK CHALLENGE

WORKBOOK

DR. CRYSTAL GREEN

How To Be Schoolgirl Skinny:
Eat Your Cake And Have Your Figure Too!
5 Week Challenge Workbook

Published by The Dream Life Foundation.

ISBN-13: 978-0615868042
ISBN-10: 0615868045

Production:
.A ELEVITA MEDIA
(elevitamedia.com)

Printed in the United States of America

First Edition

1 2 3 4 5 6 7 8 9 10

CONTENTS

INTRODUCTION   5

DOCUMENT YOUR JOURNEY   7

PRE-EVALUATION FORM   11

WEEK ONE: Getting Started   15

WEEK TWO: Let's Stay Motivated   23

WEEK THREE: Keep Moving and Grooving   27

WEEK FOUR: Arc We There Yet?   31

WEEK FIVE: And the Winner Is?   35

Appendix A: Nutrition Exam   42

References   46

About the Author   48

INTRODUCTION

This weight loss and health management five week challenge is based on the book How to Be Schoolgirl Skinny®: Eat Your Cake and Have Your Figure Too!, which is a dietary lifestyle solution created and developed by Health and Wellness Expert Dr. Crystal Green. Structured on a five week schedule to jumpstart your weight loss and health management success, this challenge applies chapters taken from the book in practical, easy, step-by-step methods that will help you master and successfully achieve your weight loss and health management goals. You can look forward to the following results if you stick to the Schoolgirl Skinny® Program.

1. Learn how to lose weight.
2. Learn why most diets and weight loss programs don't work.
3. Learn how to improve your health.
4. Learn how to improve your BMI.
5. Learn why a good night's sleep is important to your weight loss and health management.
6. Learn why exercise or some form of physical activity is essential to a healthy lifestyle.
7. Learn which supplements may be beneficial.

8. Learn the Golden Rules of Weight Management.

9. Learn how to develop a structured healthy dietary lifestyle solution.

10. Learn healthy eating habits.

11. Learn how to improve your lifestyle permanently and feel great.

Follow each week of the challenge as instructed and continue through until the fifth and final week. Then you will reach the end of the challenge but learn all of the fundamental dietary lifestyle solutions that you need to keep you on track for maintaining your weight loss goals and optimal health. Good luck and God bless as you begin your journey to a new healthy you!

DOCUMENT
YOUR
JOURNEY

T he key to your success is connected to your ability to release your thoughts, feelings, emotions, and circumstances that led up to and are directly related to your weight gain. What were the deciding factors that finally triggered your decision to take weight loss seriously? Your story is a pivotal point to your success. It indicates that you have reached a place in your life where you not only realize, but you are now ready to take ownership of your weight, your health, and your future.

You may recall my story in the Schoolgirl Skinny® book in Chapter One when my grandmother passed and two people mentioned how fat I had gotten. What I didn't mention is during the time that my weight gain had become most prominent and out of control is when I was employed for a company that I was not a fit for. I obviously was not living in my purpose-I didn't know it then, but as a certified career consultant, I recognize it now. My fat picture that is in the Schoolgirl Skinny® book is actually taken at a conference when I was employed for that company. The funny thing about that experience is that I prayed for that job. And although I learned so much while I was employed there, it was not what God had planned for me. So be careful what you ask for. You just might receive it.

The following section is a pre-evaluation form that will assist you in documenting the beginning of your journey of weight loss and health management success. You can use this workbook as your journal to document your journey. I wish you the best of luck as your triumph over the health and weight conditions that may have held you back in the past. But now know that you will soon become equipped to turn everything around for the better.

God Bless you through your journey!

PRE-EVALUATION FORM

Before you begin this journey, consider the following:

1) What led you to this point in your life that you have decided to make a life altering decision?

2) Why is this particular time different from other times that you have attempted to make a lifestyle change?

3) Who are the people that this decision will impact the most?

4) What have you specifically done to prepare for this journey that you are about to embark on?

5) If you could share one aspect about your commitment to the Schoolgirl Skinny® Program that excites you the most about your future, what would it be?

WEEK ONE
Getting Started

Week One: Getting Started

1. After you have completed the pre-evaluation form, you should have a better idea of why you are committed to the Schoolgirl Skinny® Program. This form is designed to make you think about the choices that you have made in the past and the major decision that you have recently made to jumpstart your life by incorporating a permanent dietary lifestyle solution that will change what you know about diets and unhealthy eating habits.

2. Take a before picture of yourself and place it on page 19. Write the date that you begin the Schoolgirl Skinny® Program at the top of page 19.

3. Pages 20 and 21 outline the Schoolgirl Skinny® Weight and Health Profiles. Complete them and identify your specific goals.

a. If you are unsure of your BMI, use the formula in Chapter Two of the Schoolgirl Skinny® book or use any online tool to calculate your BMI.

4. Go grocery shopping.

a. Review the grocery list in Chapter Ten and Substitution Chart in Chapter Six of the Schoolgirl Skinny® book.

b. Identify and purchase food items that will support you through this program.

5. Begin a full body detox cleansing program.

6. Track your daily progress for your journal using your cell phone, computer, notes section on your outlook, or your daily calendar. Whatever is convenient or most useful. Again, the importance of this activity is to purge your thoughts, feelings, emotions, and circumstances that led up to and are directly related to your weight gain. This form of journaling is therapeutic and will support you through your

weight loss and health management goals.

Place your *before* picture below.

Today's date is_____.

Schoolgirl Skinny® Weight Profile

GENERAL INFORMATION	CURRENT WEEK 1	PERSONAL GOAL
NAME		
AGE		
WEIGHT		
HEIGHT		
BODY WEIGHT		
BODY MASS INDEX (BMI)		

Schoolgirl Skinny® Health Profile

HEALTH CONDI-TIONS	DO YOU HAVE ANY OF THESE HEALTH CONDI-TIONS?	ARE YOU ON MEDICA-TION?	IS YOUR CONDI-TION STABLE?	GOAL
TYPE 2 DIABETES	YES NO	YES NO	YES NO	
PRE-DIABETES	YES NO	YES NO	YES NO	
HIGH BLOOD PRESSURE	YES NO	YES NO	YES NO	
HIGH CHOLES-TEROL	YES NO	YES NO	YES NO	
OBESITY	YES NO	YES NO	YES NO	
OVER-WEIGHT	YES NO	YES NO	YES NO	
HEART DISEASE	YES NO	YES NO	YES NO	

WEEK TWO

Let's Stay Motivated

Week Two: Let's Stay Motivated

1. Review Affirmations in Chapter Four.

2. Create specific affirmations that will work for you. For example, we know the reason that you started this program-to lose weight, develop a healthy lifestyle and manage your health. Therefore, your affirmations should reflect your intentions. For example, your affirmations could be...
   a. I can eat healthy and practical meals and snacks.
   b. I am at my desired weight.
   c. I am healthy, and blessed.
   d. I can now shop in my favorite section.
   Remember, you can call those things that are not as though they were. (Romans 4:17 KJV)

3. Take the Nutrition Exam in the back of this workbook (Appendix A).

4. Continue journaling your progress. You can

address specific aspects such as...

a. I was able to answer all of the nutrition questions correctly.

b. I have learned why the white stuff is not a good option for weight loss and health management.

c. I understand why it is important to include fiber and protein in my meals.

d. Now that I know how much water I should consume each day, it is easy for me to do so because I premeasure the amount, place it in a bottle and carry it with me throughout the day. And perhaps you will even consider switching to alkaline water now that your learned some of the health benefits. Refer to Golden Rule #2 in Chapter 7 of the Schoolgirl Skinny® book to learn more about the health benefits of alkaline water.

WEEK THREE

Keep Moving and Grooving

Week Three: Keep Moving and Grooving

Now that you have a great nutritional start to your dietary lifestyle solution, it's time to incorporate some fitness into the plan if you are not already doing so. For those of you who have never exercised before or do not exercise on a regular basis, as I mentioned in the How to Be Schoolgirl Skinny® book, please consult with your doctor before you begin an exercise routine. And also refer to a fitness expert when incorporating each exercise facet into your daily routine.

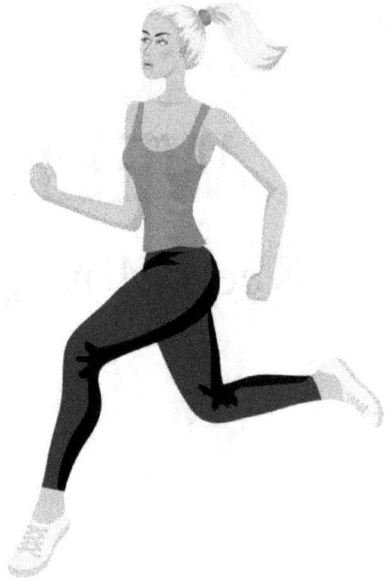

1. What physical activity do you enjoy doing?

a. Running, hiking, playing tennis, swimming,

gardening, yoga

b. Whatever you decide, that should be your primary cardio exercise.

c. Conduct a cardio workout 2-3 times a week, if you are just getting started.

d. Select 2-3 different types of cardio to work different muscle groups. You don't want your body to get used to the same exercise routine; you will notice the best results when you add variety to your workouts.

e. Start out slow, 15-20 minutes per workout, then gradually increase.

f. Each week or every two weeks, add a new exercise facet (strength training, balance, core, flexibility) to your workout routine but keep your cardio as your basic. Refer to Chapter Five.

g. If you are bored with your workout, arrange an exercise routine that can be conducted while you are watching your favorite 30 minute sitcom. Such as walking on the treadmill, using a stationary bike, stepper or elliptical.

h. Consider joining a gym or club for support and guidance.

i. Some gyms offer great workout challenges and fitness classes.

j. Get an accountability exercise partner— someone who you can work out with or at least can hold you accountable for your exercises.

WEEK FOUR

Are We There Yet?

Week Four: Are We There Yet?

Although we can receive vitamins, minerals, and nutrients from the foods that we eat, sometimes supplements can play a huge part in making up where some foods and our eating habits fall short. Review Chapter Nine and consider what are the best supplements that would be beneficial to you and why you should consider incorporating them into your daily dietary lifestyle solution process. A list of recommended supplements from Chapter Nine are noted below. Write in your journal what supplements you selected and why it was important for you to incorporate each into your daily routine.

o   Daily Multivitamin

o   Vitamin B12

o   Vitamin D3

o   PGX

o   Core Complex

o   Moringa Oleifera found in Zija Products

How Are You Sleeping?

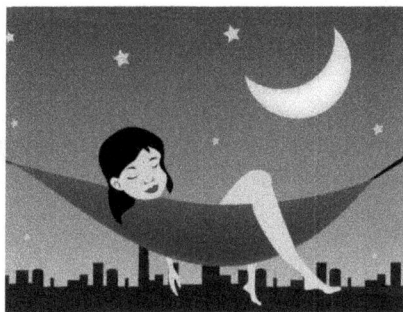

Before we end this week, let's take a look at your sleeping habits. How well are you sleeping at night? When you wake up in the morning do you feel refreshed or could you use a few more minutes or another hour or two? One of my favorite sayings is that God did not make the alarm clock-man did. Think about that for a minute. If you are not getting enough sleep at night, then not only is it impacting your metabolism so that you cannot lose weight properly, but it is also impacting your health. Refer to Chapter Eight to determine the dos and don'ts for getting your proper zzzs. Also the supplement that the body produces naturally but which can also be purchased is melatonin. However, if you are having trouble staying asleep instead of taking melatonin, you should consider magnolia bark. This herb will help you sleep through the night without waking up every few hours. You can purchase this supplement at any health food store.

WEEK FIVE

And the Winner Is?

Week Five: And the Winner Is?

And the winner is You! You have successfully completed a five week weight loss and health management challenge. You should feel terrific! Now that you understand and have completely implemented this dietary lifestyle solution based on the Schoolgirl Skinny® Program, you should be well on your way to a healthier you.

For this final section, I will share with you some final tips that you should keep in mind as you continue on your journey to success.

1. Stay encouraged: There will be times when you may not want to stick with the Schoolgirl Skinny® Program, for a number of reasons. But remember anything worth having is not going to be easy to achieve.

a. Prayer can be one of the most effective w a y s for you to continue on your path of success. Remember how much God loves you and how He desires the best for you. Take delight in the Lord, and he will give you the desires of your heart. (Psalm 37:4 NIV)

b. Check AskDrCris.com for health and wellness tips that are based on the Schoolgirl Skinny® Program.

2. Take this program one step at a time. Although you may be anxious for results, it will take time for you to receive all the benefits that you desire. Just know that as long as you are persistent, you will be blessed.

3. Review Chapter Seven in the Schoolgirl Skinny® book. Chapter Seven addresses the Golden Rules of Weight Loss Management. You should learn these rules and how to apply them in order to maintain a healthy life.

4. Complete the Follow Up Schoolgirl Skinny® Weight Profile and Follow Up Schoolgirl Skinny®

Health Profile that are noted below. The results should be encouraging to you.

5. Finally, continue documenting in your journal. Although this challenge was only for five weeks, your weight loss and health management success is for a lifetime. It will take a daily effort in order for you to continue on the path of success.

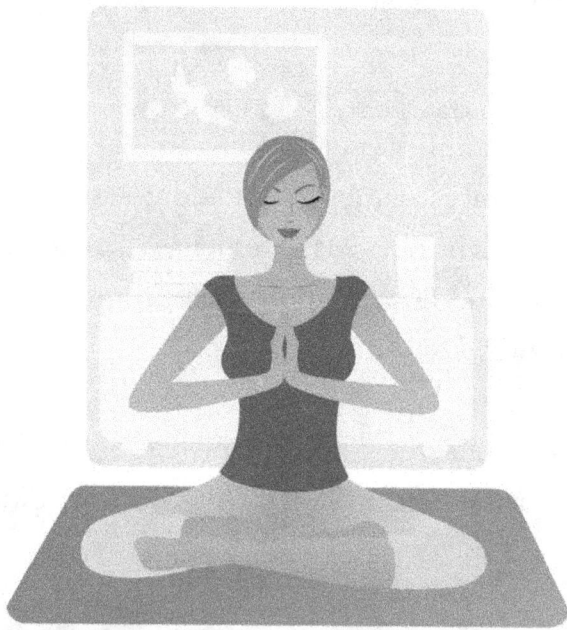

Schoolgirl Skinny® Weight Profile Follow-Up

GENERAL INFORMATION	WEEK 1	WEEK 5	PERSONAL GOAL	INDICATE IMPROVE-MENT
NAME				
AGE				
WEIGHT				
HEIGHT				
BODY WEIGHT				
BODY MASS INDEX (BMI)				

Schoolgirl Skinny® Health Profile Follow-Up

HEALTH CONDI-TIONS	HAVE ANY OF THESE HEALTH CONDI-TIONS?	ARE YOU ON MEDICA-TION?	IS YOUR CONDI-TION STABLE?	GOAL
TYPE 2 DIABETES	YES NO	YES NO	YES NO	
PRE-DIABETES	YES NO	YES NO	YES NO	
HIGH BLOOD PRESSURE	YES NO	YES NO	YES NO	
HIGH CHOLES-TEROL	YES NO	YES NO	YES NO	
OBESITY	YES NO	YES NO	YES NO	
OVER-WEIGHT	YES NO	YES NO	YES NO	
HEART DISEASE	YES NO	YES NO	YES NO	

Place your *after* picture below.

Today's date is_____.

Appendix A

Nutrition Exam

1. Fiber is not important to my daily intake.

    A. True   B. False

2. What is the "white stuff" and why should we consider not eating it?

3. I can consume as much sugar in drinks as I like and it will not impact my calorie intake or weight.

    A. True   B. False

4. Getting less than 7 hours of sleep often will not affect my weight or health.

    A. True   B. False

5. People who live in the United States do not have a problem with being overweight.

    A. True   B. False

6. Name two white flour substitutes.

7. When is the best time to eat breakfast?

8. How many glasses of water should be consumed a day on average?

9. Sources of protein are only found in meat.
          A. True   B. False

10. Can people who do not have celiac disease eat gluten free food products?

11. Where can you find the best sources of natural sugar?

12. What are some of the dietary lifestyle solutions that you learned and will implement to lose weight and stay healthy?

13. When is the best time to consumer carbohydrates?

14. Based on what you learned about supplements, which ones would fit best in your daily lifestyle and why? Choose from the list below.

a. Daily Multivitamin

b. Vitamin B12

c. Vitamin D3

d. PGX

e. Core Complex

f. Moringa Oleifera found in Zija Products

References

Week 1

How to Be Schoolgirl Skinny®: Have Your Cake and Figure Too! Chapter Ten

How to Be Schoolgirl Skinny®: Have Your Cake and Figure Too! Chapter Six

Week 2

How to Be Schoolgirl Skinny®: Have Your Cake and Figure Too! Chapter Four

Romans 4:17 KJV

Week 3

How to Be Schoolgirl Skinny®: Have Your Cake and Figure Too! Chapter Five

Week 4

How to Be Schoolgirl Skinny®: Have Your Cake and Figure Too! Chapter Nine

How to Be Schoolgirl Skinny®: Have Your Cake and Figure Too! Chapter Eight

Week 5

Psalm 37:4 NIV

How to Be Schoolgirl Skinny®: Have Your Cake and Figure Too! Chapter Seven

About the Author

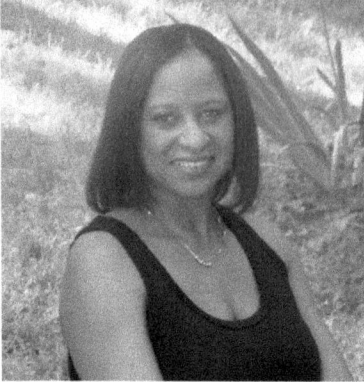

Dr. Crystal Green, Ph.D., is a Certified Career Consultant; Health/ Wellness Expert, Life Coach; and owner of Dr. Cris, the Dream Life Doctor, LLC (AskDrCris.com). She is a co-author of the *Mosaic Cross* and *Spirit of the Poet*. Her next book, *Entering Your Promised Land: Transforming Your Life to Live in Your Purpose* will challenge readers to question why they have not connected to their purpose in life sooner-and show them how to do so now.

Dr. Crystal Green is an Associate Professor for a university in Charlotte, NC and she earned the honor of appearing in Who's Who in Black Charlotte Entrepreneurs because of her dedication to the community.

www.ingramcontent.com/pod-product-compliance
Lightning Source LLC
Chambersburg PA
CBHW060656280326
41933CB00012B/2208